I'm Still Here

By Jeanette Ramirez

DEDICATION

For my children, Jordan & Juliette -
You are my reasons to keep fighting, my daily reminder of love, and the brightest light on my darkest days.

For every warrior battling an invisible illness -
May you find comfort, courage, and hope in these pages. You are never alone.

ACKNOWLEDGMENTS

This book would not exist without the love, patience, and encouragement of so many people.

To my family: thank you for walking this journey with me, for lifting me up when I felt I couldn't go on, and for loving me through every difficult day.

To my friends and community: your support, whether through a kind word, a visit, or simply standing by my side, gave me the strength to keep moving forward.

To my fellow autoimmune warriors: you inspire me every day. This book is as much yours as it is mine.

And finally, to the readers holding these pages—you are the reason I share my story. My hope is that something here touches your heart, gives you courage, and reminds you that hope still lives, even in the hardest battles.

Chapter	Title	Page #

Introduction

This is not the life I thought I'd live. I never imagined my days would be filled with medical terms I could barely pronounce, treatments that drained me, and symptoms that reshaped every part of who I am. But here I am—writing my story. Not because it's easy, but because it matters.

In 2020, after years of unexplained symptoms and constant frustration, I was officially diagnosed with scleroderma, a rare and complex autoimmune disease. But my journey didn't start there. My body had been speaking in whispers for a long time—through fatigue, pain, stiffness, digestive issues, and more. The problem was no one was really listening. Not even me at times.

Scleroderma, which literally means "hard skin," is so much more than skin deep. It can affect organs, joints, blood vessels, and every corner of your life—physically, emotionally, and spiritually. In my case, it's part of a broader diagnosis: Mixed Connective Tissue Disease, a rare overlap of autoimmune conditions that's often invisible to others but never to me.

This book isn't just about the pain. It's about the fight.

It's about losing parts of yourself and still finding the strength to show up anyway.
It's about being doubted, dismissed, and still choosing to believe in your worth.
It's about learning to live with what feels unbearable—and somehow making space for joy.

I've created this for the people who live with chronic illness, for those newly diagnosed and desperately Googling symptoms at 2 a.m., and for the friends, family, and caretakers who want to understand but don't always know how. I also wrote it for the version of me who needed a voice like this years ago—raw, honest, and unfiltered.

This isn't a medical guide. It's a human story.
One that I hope brings awareness, validation, and maybe even healing.

You are not alone.
And I'm so glad you're here.

~ Jeanette ~

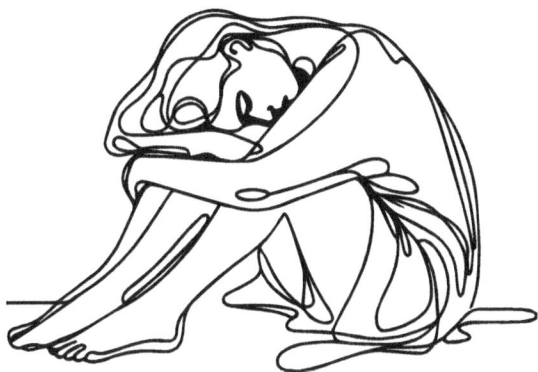

Chapter 1: Something's Not Right

Before the name, before the diagnosis, there was just...
something.

At first, it was easy to dismiss.

It started small, almost quietly. I blamed stress, long days, or just getting older. But then the signs became louder. It wasn't just that I was tired. It was a bone-deep exhaustion that sleep couldn't fix. It wasn't just that my hands were cold—it was that they'd turn white and numb, even when the weather was fine. I'd get odd digestive flare-ups, strange joint pain, and random swelling that had no explanation.

Then the fatigue came.

Not just tired. Not "I stayed up too late" tired. This was the kind of fatigue that crawled into my bones.

I would rest, nap, sleep all night - and still wake up feeling like I ran a marathon in my dreams.

I tried to power through. I was a mother, a worker, a woman with responsibilities. There was no time to fall apart. But inside, I knew something was shifting. Something just wasn't right.

It's an eerie thing - to live in a body that's screaming at you, while the rest of the world insists it is whispering.

I began to feel like I was living in two realities: the one where I looked fine, smiled, and went about my day... and the one where I was slowly falling apart on the inside.

My body was whispering that something was wrong, and that whisper turned into a scream.

Deep down, I knew.
Something was off.

The hardest part in those early days wasn't the symptoms—it was the confusion. I bounced from appointment to appointment, trying to explain what I was feeling. Doctors nodded politely, ordered bloodwork, and handed me reassurances that didn't match the reality of my pain.

I remember sitting in one of those early appointments clutching my handwritten symptom list. I had rehearsed it in my head a dozen times. When it was my turn, I poured everything out— the swelling, the fatigue, the aches, and the joint pain. The doctor skimmed my labs, glanced up at me, and said, "Everything looks fine. You're probably just stressed."

I smiled weakly and nodded, but walking out of that office, I felt invisible. My body was screaming, but no one was listening.

I went to several other doctors.

A lot of them.

Each time hoping this one would finally take me seriously. Each time walking away with a shrug, a prescription that didn't help, or worse—being told it was "just anxiety."
You start to wonder if you're imagining things.
You start to feel crazy.

But I wasn't crazy. I was sick.
And my body had been trying to tell me that for a long time.

That was the beginning of my journey—the moment I realized I was entering a fight I didn't fully understand yet. Looking back, those early signs were the opening chapter of a story that would change my life forever.

The scariest part? I had no name for what I was experiencing. No clear answer. No direction. Just a body that was betraying me in slow motion. And a system that didn't seem to be in any rush to catch me.

One of the hardest parts of chronic illness is the waiting.
The not knowing.
The being told it's *probably nothing* when you know

it's something.

There's a grief that starts long before the diagnosis. A mourning of the life you had, of the trust you once had in your body, and the quiet, creeping fear that maybe you'll never feel "normal" again.

But even then—even in the confusion and the frustration—there was a part of me that held on.
Because when your body is fighting a battle that no one else can see, **you learn to become your own advocate.**

I didn't know then that I'd be diagnosed with a rare disease.
I didn't know that it would come with pain, procedures, and a lifetime of management.

But I did know this:
Something was not right.
Deep down, I knew it had a name - I just hadn't met it yet.
And I wasn't going to stop until I found out what it was.

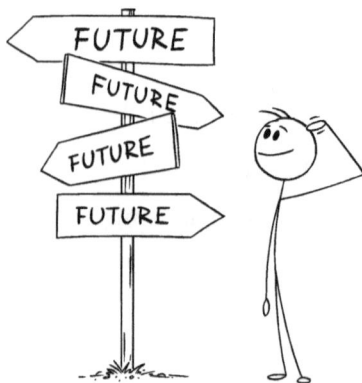

Chapter 2: The Diagnosis That Changed Everything

It had a name. But that didn't make it any less terrifying.

When the word *scleroderma* finally entered my life, it didn't come as a relief—it came as a shock. Instead, it felt like being handed a life sentence without parole.

After years of bouncing from specialist to specialist, enduring bloodwork, scans, scopes, and endless dead ends, I was finally given a name for what was happening to my body. But nothing could have prepared me for what that name meant.

The weeks (turned into years) that followed were a blur of blood work, referrals, specialists, online rabbit holes, and late-night tears. I learned that scleroderma wasn't just about skin—it could affect the lungs, heart, kidneys, and digestive system. I learned how rare it was, and how little most people—even doctors—understood about it.

It wasn't a simple fix or a one-pill solution. It was a rare, chronic, autoimmune disease. One that affects the connective tissue—tightening the skin, damaging internal organs, and creating inflammation throughout the body. In my case, it was part of a larger diagnosis: Mixed Connective Tissue Disease (MCTD), a blend of several autoimmune conditions —scleroderma being one of the most aggressive among them.

I remember the day I heard the word scleroderma, my world shifted. Up until then, I had clung to the hope that maybe this was something simple— something that could be fixed with rest, vitamins, or a short course of treatment. But when the doctor spoke, that hope slipped away.

I sat there trying to process what the doctor was saying, but the words felt like they were coming through water.

Hard skin.
Raynaud's.
Esophageal dysmotility.
Pulmonary complications.
No cure.
No cure.
NO CURE?

That one hit the hardest.

I nodded and asked questions, pretending to process what she was saying. Inside, though, I was spiraling. *Scleroderma.* I had never even heard of it before. How could this strange, complicated word suddenly define my future?

I left the office gripping my paperwork so tightly my knuckles turned white. When I got into my car, I couldn't turn the key. My hands shook as I held the steering wheel, and the tears came hard and fast. I cried for the diagnosis, yes, but also for the life I thought I'd have—the one that now seemed to be slipping away.

That moment marked the dividing line in my life: before I knew, and after. Nothing would ever be the same again.

Up until then, I had been waiting for the doctor who would finally give me something to make it all go away. I believed if I just got the right answer, I could go back to who I was before. But this diagnosis didn't offer that.

Instead, it offered the reality that I would be living with this for the rest of my life.

My first instinct was denial. Maybe they were wrong. Maybe it was a mistake.
But the test results didn't lie.
And neither did my body. I had just been hoping for a different truth.

What followed was a whirlwind—more tests, more doctors, more medical language I had to Google. I had to learn a whole new vocabulary just to understand what was happening inside me.

Then came the questions:

What does this mean for my future?
Will I end up in a wheelchair?
Will I lose my independence?
Will anyone understand what I'm going through?

And perhaps the hardest one:
Why **me?**

I didn't get an answer to that. Most of us don't.
But in time, I stopped asking why and started asking *how.*

How do I live with this?
How do I still find purpose?
How do I fight without losing myself?

Because even though the diagnosis changed everything, it also gave me something I didn't expect...direction.

Now I had a name.
Now I could learn.
Now I could prepare, advocate, and build a life around truth instead of confusion.

Scleroderma didn't just change the trajectory of my health—it changed the way I saw the world, and more importantly, how I saw myself. I wasn't weak. I was navigating something most people couldn't even imagine.

And slowly, I began to realize that this diagnosis—while devastating—was also a doorway.
Not to an ending, but to a new version of my life.

Some told me I was lucky it wasn't worse.
Some told me to stay positive.
But no one told me how to *live* with it.

I tried to act normal. I went to work. I made dinner. I smiled at my kids. But inside, I was unraveling. Fear wrapped around me like a second skin—tight, suffocating, always there.

The hardest part? I didn't look sick.

People couldn't see the war going on inside my body. So, they assumed I was fine. I started to feel like I was faking wellness just to keep others comfortable.

But I wasn't okay.

I was terrified.

And I was completely, completely alone.

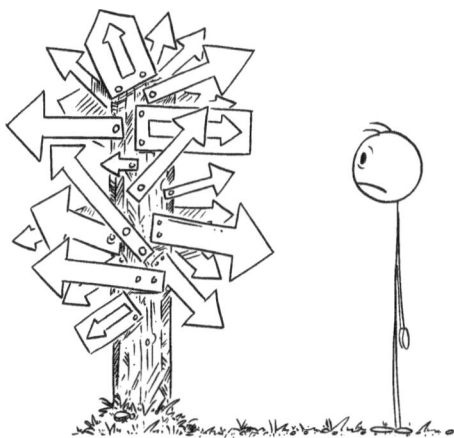

Chapter 3: Living in a Body That's Changing

What do you do when the body you've always known starts to feel like a stranger?

One of the cruelest parts of scleroderma is how it changes you from the inside out—often without warning and without permission.

Some days, it feels like I've been evicted from my own body.

Like I woke up one day and found that someone else had taken over—and left me in a body that no longer listens to me.

After the diagnosis, I started to notice changes I had been ignoring before. My body felt foreign to me, as if I was slowly being reshaped from the inside out.

It started with my hands. They'd swell without reason and feel tight like rubber bands stretched to the limit. Simple things—like buttoning clothes, opening jars, or even texting—became frustrating. Some days, they seemed impossible.

Then came the cold intolerances. I'd feel a chill in my fingers and toes even on warm days. Raynaud's phenomenon—one of scleroderma's many companions—would leave my fingers ghost white, purple, or bright red, painfully stiff and numb. The cold became my enemy, and winter stopped being just a season. It became a trigger.

Over time, it wasn't just my hands. My face changed. My skin lost elasticity. The mirror started showing a version of me I didn't quite recognize.

But the changes that were *invisible* to others? Those were the ones that cut the deepest.

I started having trouble swallowing. At meals, food would get stuck halfway down. Swallowing water burned.

My esophagus—like much of my body—was stiffening. I had to sit up after every meal and avoid certain foods. I couldn't eat spicy food, greasy food, or sometimes even solid food. The joy of eating—gone.

Eventually it got to the point where I had to go in for regular procedures to have it stretched. That's not something you expect to hear in your 40s.

I dealt with joint pain that would flare without warning, stomach issues that made planning anything risky, and a fatigue so consuming it felt like my body was moving through wet cement.

But the most haunting change was the fatigue.

Previously, I was told I had an "ungodly" amount of energy—people joked that I never stopped moving. Now, even the simplest tasks can leave me drained, like I've run a marathon I never signed up for. It's not just tiredness; it's a bone-deep exhaustion that no amount of rest seems to cure.

It's hard to explain the kind of exhaustion that scleroderma brings. It's not tired. It's not sleepy. It's *cell-deep depletion*. I'd lie in bed for hours, unable to move, just blinking and breathing.

Friends would say, *"You look so good!"* but all I saw was a stranger trying to hold herself together.

The invisibility is one of the cruelest parts.
Because while I was dealing with daily body betrayal, people still expected me to function. Smile. Work. Show up.
And I did. I still do.
But it comes at a cost.

I've had to become hyper-aware of every ache, every new sensation, every subtle shift. I learned to listen carefully because I don't get the luxury of ignoring it anymore.

Yes, my body is changing. And yes, it hurts.
But with every shift, I've also learned how strong I

really am.

Not strong in the "I've got this all figured out" way.
Strong in the "I got out of bed today even though my body didn't want to move" way.
Strong in the "I still showed up" way.

It wasn't just physical; it was emotional, too. Every new limitation was another reminder that my body was no longer the same. I grieved those losses silently, not wanting to burden the people around me, but inside I was constantly wrestling with the reality of change.

Scleroderma didn't just alter my body—it altered my sense of self. I had to learn, day by day, how to live inside this changing shell, and how to accept that strength now looked different than it once did.

I didn't ask for this body. But I'm learning to live with it.

Some days it feels like war.
Some days it feels like peace.
But every day, it's mine.

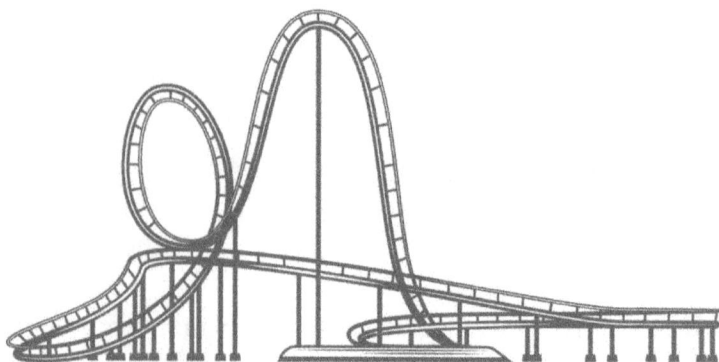

Chapter 4: The Emotional Rollercoaster

This disease doesn't just affect the body—it wrecks the heart, the mind, and the spirit.

It wraps its hands around your mental health and squeezes.

Nobody talks enough about the emotional side of chronic illness.

Yes, there's pain. Yes, there are hospital visits, medications, and symptoms.
But beneath all that is something heavier—a constant inner storm most people never see.

When I was first diagnosed, I felt everything all at once: relief, fear, anger, confusion. I finally had a name for what was happening, but that name came with a weight I wasn't ready for. And no one hands you a guide on how to emotionally survive something that never ends.

Some days, I feel strong. Other days, I feel shattered.

And there's a unique kind of grief that comes with chronic illness. You grieve your old life, your old body, your old energy. You mourn routines you used to take for granted—waking up without pain, running errands without exhaustion, eating without anxiety. It's a quiet kind of grief, the kind that lives in your chest and doesn't let up.

And then there's the guilt.

The guilt of canceling plans.
The guilt of feeling like a burden.
The guilt of being "unreliable" in a world that expects consistency.

Even when people say, *"Take care of yourself,"* part of

me still hears, *"You're letting them down."*

The truth is, I miss showing up for others the way I used to.
I *miss* being the dependable one.
I *miss* the me who didn't always have to explain or justify her pain.

But even worse than guilt is isolation.

People check in—for a while. Then the texts slow down. The invites stop. And suddenly, you're watching life happen from the sidelines, wondering if anyone even remembers the version of you that used to dance at parties or stay out late or go on spontaneous road trips. Now everything needs to be planned around energy levels, flare risks, medications, and appointments.

It's lonely.
Even when you're surrounded by people, it's lonely.

And then there's the fear.

Fear of the unknown.

Fear of the disease progression.
Fear of losing independence.

Every new symptom feels like a landmine. Every doctor appointment brings anxiety. Every "we found something" threatens to derail months of hard-won stability.

I've broken down in bathrooms. In parking lots. In the middle of folding laundry.
I've cried quietly during conversations, smiling while my heart cracked open.

The worst part is pretending.

Pretending to be okay so people don't worry.
Pretending I'm not upset when someone cancels because they're concerned about my weakened immune system.
Pretending that it doesn't hurt when friends disappear because my life is no longer convenient.

But with all that pain came a quiet strength.

I've learned to sit with the emotions instead of

running from them.

I've learned that it's okay to be angry.
It's okay to cry.
It's okay to scream into a pillow or write in a journal or say, "this is unfair."

Because it *is* unfair.

And at the same time, I've learned how powerful I can be in my own sadness. I've learned how to feel everything and still move forward.

Some days I fall apart.
Some days I put myself back together.
Both are valid. Both are part of this life.

I started therapy. I opened up online. I found support groups. I started writing—not for anyone else, just for me. The more I shared, the less alone I felt. And slowly, the emotional weight became something I could carry—not every day, not easily—but I carried it.

Scleroderma didn't just challenge my body. It cracked

open my heart.

And what's come out hasn't just been grief or rage—it's also been growth, compassion, patience, and empathy.

Chronic illness is not just a physical battle—it's also an emotional one. My body wasn't the only thing changing; my heart and mind were too.

Some days, I felt strong and ready to fight. Other days, I felt like I was drowning. The unpredictability was its own kind of torture—never knowing if I'd wake up with energy or if the day would end in tears.

There were moments of deep anger. Anger at my body for betraying me, anger at doctors for not having answers, anger at the universe for handing me something I never asked for. There were also moments of despair, when I wondered what kind of future I really had left.

One night, I sat in the dark living room long after everyone else had gone to bed. My body ached from head to toe, and my mind was racing. I pressed my fists into my eyes and whispered, "I can't do this anymore." The silence answered back, but somehow, I found myself breathing again, standing again, showing up again the next day. That cycle became familiar— the rise and fall of emotions, the breaking and rebuilding.

This emotional rollercoaster may not end. But I've learned to hold on, to ride the dips, to breathe through the twists. And when I can, I reach out my hand to someone else riding their own version of this disease.

Because while this journey is mine, it was never meant to be walked alone.

I'm still on this rollercoaster.

There are high points—moments of joy, days of energy, connection, growth.

There are low points—flares, fatigue, fear, frustration.

But I ride them all now with open eyes.
Because I may not control this ride, but I *am* holding the wheel.

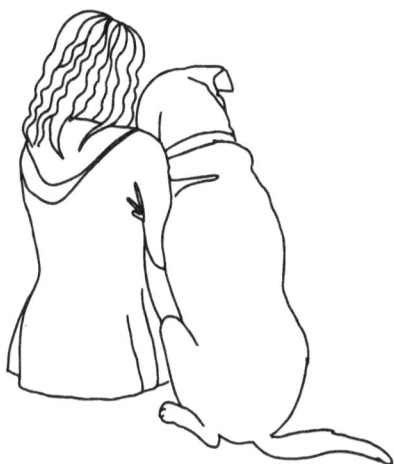

Chapter 5: The Grieving Process No One Talks About

When I was first diagnosed, no one ever told me I would go through a grieving process. Not grief in the way people usually think of it—not the loss of a loved one—but the loss of myself, the life I once had, and the future I thought I knew.

I didn't recognize it at the time. I just thought I was overwhelmed, exhausted, angry, and sad. I thought I was "failing" at handling my illness. What I didn't realize was that I was moving through the stages of grief: denial, anger, bargaining, depression, and eventually, acceptance.

Denial was the quiet voice that told me, *"Maybe they're wrong. Maybe it's not really scleroderma."* It was me pushing through, pretending I could still do everything the same way, even when my body screamed otherwise.

Anger came in waves. Anger at doctors, at my body, at God, at the unfairness of it all. It wasn't polite or pretty—it was raw and heavy, and sometimes it scared me.

Bargaining showed up in whispered promises: *"If I just eat better, if I just exercise more, if I just take all these medications… maybe this will go away."* I thought I could outsmart the disease, trade in effort for healing.

Depression crept in quietly. It looked like isolation, endless fatigue, and the feeling that no one understood what I was carrying. Some days it looked like tears; other days it looked like numbness.

Acceptance didn't come overnight. It didn't even come in a neat, final package. Acceptance for me has been messy. It's about finding peace in the fact that my body is different now, that my life is different, but also realizing I am still *me*. That there is still joy, laughter, love, and purpose.

I wish someone had told me I was grieving, because maybe then I would have been kinder to myself in the beginning. Maybe I wouldn't have felt so lost inside emotions that felt unpredictable and out of control.

So, if you're reading this and you've just been diagnosed—please hear me: what you're feeling is grief, and it's okay. You are mourning the life you had, and that is natural. Give yourself permission to feel it, to move through it at your own pace, and to know that acceptance doesn't mean giving up. It means learning to live again, differently, but still beautifully.

No one prepared me for the grief.

When people think of grief, they think of death, of funerals, of losing someone you love. But chronic illness carries its own kind of grief—the grief of losing the life you thought you'd have.

I grieved quietly, often without even recognizing it. I grieved the body I once lived in, the one that could run, dance, and move freely without pain. I grieved the ease of waking up and not having to calculate how much energy the day would demand. I grieved the future I had imagined, one that now felt uncertain and out of reach.

One afternoon, I found myself staring at an old photo—me on the beach, hair blowing in the wind, smiling without effort, barefoot in the sand. My chest tightened as tears spilled over. I missed that girl. I missed her freedom. I wasn't just missing a moment in time; I was mourning a version of myself that no longer existed.

And like all grief, it came in waves. Some days I felt acceptance. Other days I felt denial, anger, or deep sadness. The cycle repeated itself over, and over again, and I learned that healing doesn't mean the grief disappears—it just changes shape.

This grieving process is something I wish more people understood. Because when you live with chronic illness, you don't just lose health—you lose certainty, spontaneity, and parts of your identity. But with that loss also comes a chance to rebuild, to discover strength you never knew you had, and to create a new life within the one you never asked for.

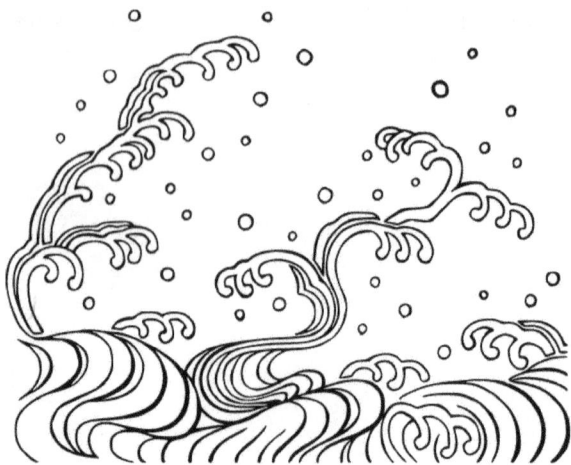

Chapter 6: Riding the Waves of Emotion

There are mornings when I wake up determined to conquer the day, and there are mornings when the weight of everything presses so hard against my chest that I wonder how I will even make it to the kitchen. Living with chronic illness is like riding waves that never stop coming. Some are small and gentle, lifting me with a reminder that joy still exists. Others are powerful and relentless, crashing over me and leaving me gasping for breath.

In the beginning, I didn't understand how much space this illness would take in my heart and mind. I thought it was just about the physical pain—the stiffness, the swelling, the fatigue. But over time, I realized the emotional toll is just as consuming, if not heavier. It's the uncertainty. It's the grief for the life I used to have. It's the guilt of canceling plans again. It's the fear of the unknown.

One night, I lay awake, staring at the ceiling, replaying the words of yet another doctor who had no answers. My mind spun with questions—Will I ever feel normal again? Will my children remember me as the mom who always had to rest? Will I keep getting worse? The questions pulled me under like riptides. But then, in the silence, I heard laughter from the next room—my daughter giggling at a silly video before bed. That sound broke through the storm inside me. It reminded me that joy still lives here, even when pain tries to drown it out.

What made it worse was the waves come crashing in during moments I least expected.

I remember being at work behind the bar, my hands aching from Raynaud's, barely able to twist open a bottle. I wanted to cry from frustration. Then a customer cracked a joke so ridiculous I burst out laughing. For a few seconds, the pain didn't own me. That moment became a reminder that I could still find light, even in places I didn't go looking for it.

These waves will never stop. But I've learned I don't always have to fight them. Sometimes I let them carry me. Sometimes I dive beneath and wait for them to pass. And sometimes I ride them, shaky but determined, knowing that no matter how high or low they take me, I am still moving forward.

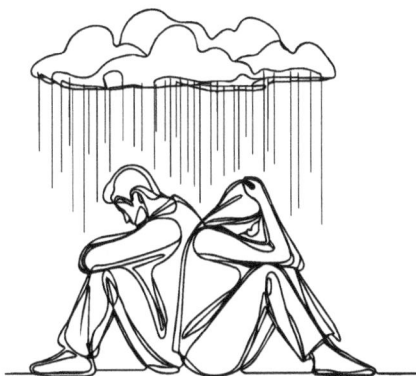

Chapter 7: More Than Just Scleroderma (MCTD)

When people hear that I have scleroderma, they often stop listening there. It's a complicated word, a rare disease, and most people can't imagine living with it. But what they don't realize is that scleroderma is only one piece of my story.

My true diagnosis is something called **Mixed Connective Tissue Disease (MCTD)**. It's not a single illness, but an overlap of several autoimmune diseases. In other words, my body didn't choose just one way to attack itself—it chose many.

Each condition adds its own challenges:

Scleroderma tightens my skin and affects my organs, making simple movements difficult and even my breathing feel restricted at times.

Lupus brings inflammation that can strike anywhere—joints, skin, even organs—most of the times with little warning.

Rheumatoid Arthritis locks my joints in pain, making tasks like tying shoes or opening a jar feel like monumental efforts.

Gastroparesis slows down my digestion, leaving food sitting in my stomach for hours instead of moving through normally. Eating becomes complicated: too much, and I feel painfully bloated; too little, and I'm weak and malnourished. Sometimes, even the smell of food makes me nauseous. The joy of sharing meals is replaced with calculations about what my body might tolerate today.

Barrett's Esophagus is another unwelcome guest —caused by years of acid reflux burning my esophagus. It's more than just heartburn; it's a constant fire in my chest, a risk factor for cancer, and another reminder that my body is fighting battles on the inside I can't always feel right away.

Raynaud's Phenomenon turns my fingers and toes ghostly white, blue, or red when exposed to cold or even mild stress. The pain can feel like knives of ice stabbing through my hands.

Once, I was in the grocery store when Raynaud's hit. My fingers went ghostly white and stiff as I held the cart. The pain was sharp, stabbing, as though ice had replaced my blood. I tried to push through, but eventually I abandoned the cart and walked out empty-handed. Something as ordinary as shopping for groceries had been stolen from me.

Epstein–Barr Virus (EBV), which is like mononucleosis, lingers in my system like an unwelcome shadow. Many people recover from mono and move on, but for me, EBV seems to fuel autoimmune flares, dragging me back into cycles of fatigue, swollen glands, and body aches whenever my immune system dips.

The overlap of all these conditions doesn't just add

symptoms—it multiplies them. Some days it feels like my body is spinning a roulette wheel, and I never know which illness will show up strongest.

MCTD isn't just a medical term on my chart. It's the reason why my life looks different than it used to. It's the reason I had to rebuild routines, redefine strength, and relearn who I am. It's complicated, messy, and unpredictable—but it's also part of my reality. And naming it gave me one thing I desperately needed: clarity.

The hardest part? These conditions don't take turns. They pile on top of each other. Some days I can't tell where the lupus ends, and the scleroderma begins. Other days it feels like they're working together, ganging up on me all at once.

Trying to explain this to others is almost impossible. If I say I have scleroderma, people nod politely. If I list everything—scleroderma, lupus, rheumatoid arthritis, gastroparesis, Barrett's esophagus, and more —they look at me like I'm exaggerating. Like no one could possibly be carrying all of that at once. But I am. Every single day.

What keeps me grounded is knowing that sharing the full truth matters. Because there are others out there with MCTD, living with their own combination of overlapping diseases, wondering if anyone else understands. To them, I want to say: *Yes. I see you. I am you.*

Living with MCTD isn't just about medical challenges —it's about identity. It forces me to redefine what "healthy" means, what "normal" looks like, and what "strength" feels like. It's about waking up every day not knowing which version of my body I'll get and learning to live with that unpredictability.

I used to think I was fighting one battle. But the truth is, I'm navigating a war on multiple fronts. And yet, here I am—still living, still fighting, still finding joy. Not because it's easy, but because life is still worth every ounce of the fight.

A Day in the Life

To give you an idea of what MCTD feels like in real life, let me take you through one ordinary morning.

I open my eyes before sunrise, but I don't wake up refreshed. My body feels heavy, like I'm pinned to the mattress by invisible weights. My hands are stiff, curled slightly, and I have to massage them gently just to flex my fingers. The first victory of the day is getting them to bend enough to hold my phone.

When I finally sit up, acid burns the back of my throat. Barrett's esophagus reminds me that I can't just roll out of bed—I need to sit upright slowly, sip water carefully, and avoid eating for at least an hour.

My stomach churns from gastroparesis, and even though I'm hungry, I know breakfast will be complicated.

I make it to the kitchen, shuffling because my knees ache from rheumatoid arthritis. I reach for a coffee mug, and pain shoots through my wrists. I pause, breathe, and pick it up with both hands like it's made of glass. Even holding a cup requires strategy.

By mid-morning, lupus has already joined the party. My skin feels sensitive, like I've been sunburned from the inside, out. My joints swell and ache, and the fatigue drapes over me like a thick blanket I can't push off.

And yet—life goes on. I answer messages. I push through chores. I put on a smile for the people who need to see it, even while my body is silently screaming.

This is the reality of MCTD. It's not just one illness. It's layers of illness, stacked and tangled, demanding energy and resilience I never knew I had.

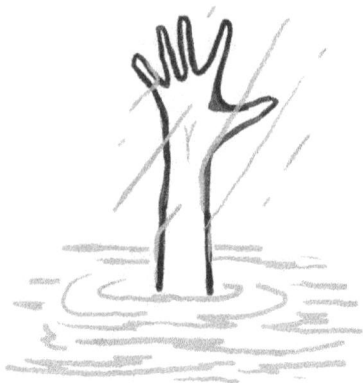

Chapter 8: Drowning in Doctors, Drowning in Pills

At one point, managing my illness felt less like living and more like existing as a professional patient. My calendar was filled with appointments—one, two, even three in a single week. Each visit brought new lab slips, more procedures, and another prescription to add to the growing line of pill bottles on my nightstand.

Every week meant waiting rooms, fluorescent lights, and explaining my symptoms repeatedly to new faces. I became fluent in medical jargon, but no matter how many tests they ran, one thing stayed the same: my pain. And ironically, none of the 22 pills I swallowed every single day were for that.

Yes, twenty-two pills. Every morning and night, I lined them up like soldiers. Alongside them was a weekly methotrexate injection—a chemo-level drug that left me weak and nauseated. And then came the monthly infusion, a ritual of poking and prodding because nurses could never find a good vein. By the time they finally got the IV started, I was already exhausted. Before the treatment even began.

One infusion day, I sat in the chair for over an hour while two nurses tried repeatedly to find a vein. My arms were covered in fresh bruises and old ones, evidence of every failed attempt. By the time the medication finally began dripping into me, I felt less like a person and more like a pin cushion.

It consumed my life. Driving to appointments, sitting in waiting rooms, following up with pharmacies, fighting with insurances. My body was exhausted, but my spirit was even more worn down. I couldn't escape the feeling that instead of treating me, the system was simply piling more, and more onto me.

The hardest part was realizing that these medications were supposed to "prolong my life." That's what I was told over, and over again. But at what cost? My days weren't being lived—they were being managed. My calendar wasn't filled with memories or moments; it was filled with appointments. I wasn't surviving, I was *existing*. And deep down, I started to question: *What if they're not prolonging my life at all? What if they're making me worse?*

I began to question everything. Who were these doctors to tell me they were extending my life? How could they know? Anyone—me, them, you—can be gone tomorrow in a freak accident. And if that's true, why was I spending all my *todays* in hospitals, drs offices, and pharmacies, chained to medications that weren't even easing my worst complaint: the pain?

I reached a breaking point.

So, I made a choice that scared even me.

Slowly, carefully, I began weaning myself off the mountain of medications. It wasn't easy—my body had become dependent on them, and withdrawal was brutal. It rebelled. It chose violence.

I lost overnthirty pounds. For three or four months, I

struggled to eat. Whatever I was able to consume, quickly left my body. It was ruthless.

The hunger, the nausea, the weakness—it nearly broke me. But I couldn't keep drowning in pills that weren't helping.

I didn't walk away from every medication. I kept the essentials—my stomach meds, (because gut health is essential when you're fighting autoimmune disease), allergy pills, and a few other things I truly needed. But I stopped giving away all my time, money, and energy to treatments that were robbing me of the very life they claimed to preserve.

That decision didn't "fix" me. I am still in pain every day. But for the first time, I felt like I had reclaimed a piece of control. I wasn't just a passive patient anymore, swallowed by appointments and prescriptions. I was a person again, *choosing* how to live my life.

Then something shifted. As the drugs left my system, so did some of the fog. I wasn't better—but I felt clearer. My life was no longer dictated by pill bottles and appointment reminders.

I know some people won't agree with my choice. I know doctors may shake their heads. But this is my body, my life, and my fight. And I chose to reclaim it.

Because the truth is, living longer means nothing if you're not really *living*.

Journal Entries from the Breaking Point

May 3

Another infusion day. Three nurses, five attempts, two bruises later—they finally got a vein. I cried in the bathroom stall after because I'm just so tired of being a pincushion.

August 15

Pill bottles line my nightstand like trophies I never wanted. TWENTY TWO a day. My body feels poisoned, yet the pain still rages. None of these are helping me.

October 2

Sitting in the care after a Dr appointment and started to wonder: What if I just stop? The thought terrified me but also gave me a strange sense of peace.

January 10

Three months off most of the meds. Down 30 pounds. I can barely eat. I don't feel "better," but I feel like I'm finally in charge of my own body again.

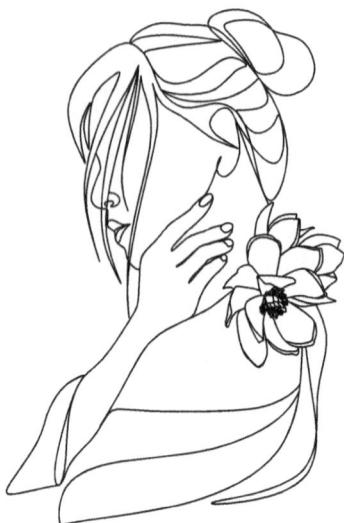

Chapter 9: What Healing Looks Like for Me

For a long time, I thought healing meant a cure. I thought it meant going back to the person I was before—the woman who could juggle kids, work, errands, and still have energy left at the end of the day. But chronic illness changes that definition. Healing isn't about going back. For me, it's about learning to move forward in a body that doesn't always cooperate.

Healing looks different now. It looks like balance. It looks like listening to my body instead of ignoring it. Some days, it's giving myself permission to rest without guilt. Other days, it's pushing through just enough to remind myself that I can still move, still live, still show up for the things and people I love.

I've experimented with countless approaches. Doctors prescribed medications that I still use sparingly, but I also discovered that gut health was central to how I feel. Healing looks like paying attention to what foods my body tolerates, learning to prepare meals slowly and intentionally, celebrating the days I can actually enjoy what's on my plate.

I remember the first time I tried eliminating certain foods to help with my gastroparesis. It felt impossible at first—restricting, frustrating—but then I noticed my stomach pain easing ever so slightly. It wasn't a miracle, but it was something. That small change gave me hope that healing can come in pieces, not in grand fixes.

Sometimes, healing is mental and spiritual. It's stepping outside on a hard day, letting the sun hit my face, and reminding myself that I am still alive. It's journaling, releasing the fears swirling inside my head. It's laughing with my kids even when my body aches, because joy is its own kind of medicine.

Healing, for me, isn't about erasing illness. It's about reclaiming pieces of myself in the middle of it.

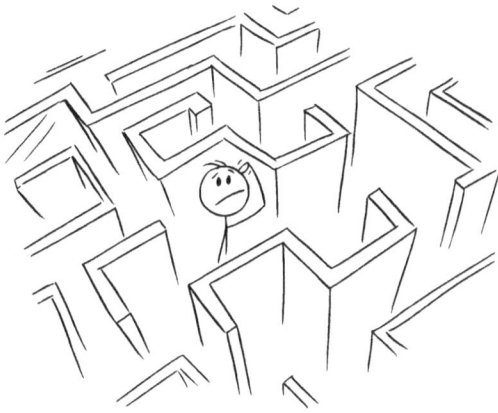

Chapter 10: Managing the Medical Maze

If you ever want to learn the true meaning of "exhaustion," try being your own case manager while chronically ill.

It isn't just the disease itself that consumes your energy—it's the endless logistics of managing it.

Managing this disease means managing people: primary doctors, specialists, nurses, lab techs, schedulers, pharmacists, insurance reps, and sometimes even the billing department. It means learning a new language—one filled with acronyms, test codes, side effects, and treatment plans.

No one tells you when you're diagnosed that you become the one holding all the strings together. No one hands you a roadmap.

Every new symptom means a new referral. Every new referral means a new intake form, another waitlist, another hour explaining your story to someone who just skimmed your chart and likely doesn't really understand anyway.

A Life of Appointments

My weeks blurred into a cycle of appointments. rheumatologist on Monday, gastroenterologist on Wednesday, pulmonologist the week after that, infusion center once a month. Each specialist wanted more blood work, more scans, more follow-ups. And because nothing about autoimmune disease is simple, one appointment always created the need for another.

Some weeks, I spent more time in waiting rooms than I did at home. The same stack of intake forms, the same cold exam tables, the same rehearsed explanation of my symptoms. I became a professional patient—an identity I never wanted.

The Day I Played Ping-Pong with My Health

One morning, I had an early appointment with my gastroenterologist. After hours of waiting, he suggested I "check in" with my rheumatologist for some labs to make sure nothing else was going on. That same day, I drove across town to squeeze into a last-minute slot with my rheumatologist. By the time I finally sat in her office, my body was screaming from fatigue, and I was fighting back tears. I left with more lab slips in my hand than answers in my head.

Tests, Procedures, and More Tests

There were scopes that left me sore, CT scans that left me anxious, and endless vials of blood drawn until my veins hardened with scar tissue. Even routine labs were exhausting. And behind every test was a wait—for results, for callbacks, for the next round of "we just need a little more information."

It was consuming—not just physically, but mentally

61

and emotionally. My life wasn't just interrupted by my illness; it was swallowed by the process of managing it.

Insurance Denial #17

I remember once being told I needed a specific test before adjusting a medication. My doctor ordered it, but insurance denied it—twice. I spent hours on the phone, re-explaining my condition to people who couldn't pronounce it, let alone understand it. By the time the test was approved weeks later, the flare I needed it for had already passed. I didn't get care—I got paperwork.

The Paperwork and Phone Calls

What people rarely talk about is the paperwork. Insurance approvals, denials, prior authorizations, medical records requests—it was a second job I never applied for. I spent hours on the phone with insurance companies, re-explaining things they already had in their files, being transferred from department to department.

And always, the money. Copays, lab bills, hospital charges, prescription costs. Even with insurance, the financial burden of being sick was staggering.

The Binder

I carried a thick binder with me everywhere—test results, medication lists, doctor notes, discharge papers. I was the middleman between my own specialists. If I didn't lug that binder to every appointment, something critical would be "missing from the chart." I learned quickly that if I didn't advocate for myself, no one else was connecting the dots.

Becoming My Own Case Manager

Eventually, I realized something: no one was coordinating my care but me. The specialists didn't always talk to each other. The burden of connecting the dots fell squarely on my shoulders. If I didn't track my medications, my labs, my symptoms, and my referrals, things slipped through the cracks.

So, I became my own case manager—my own

advocate. I kept binders of paperwork, journals of symptoms, spreadsheets of medications. I learned to ask hard questions. I learned to say, "That doesn't make sense—explain it again."

But that constant vigilance came at a price. The stress of staying on top of it all was its own trigger, fueling my symptoms and worsening my health.

The Exhaustion of the Maze

There were days I left appointments in tears, not from what the doctor said, but from the sheer weight of it all. The running, the scheduling, the sitting, the waiting, the explaining, the bills—it never ended.

It felt like my entire existence had been reduced to a full-time job of being sick. And in that maze of appointments, tests, and procedures, it was easy to lose sight of *myself*.

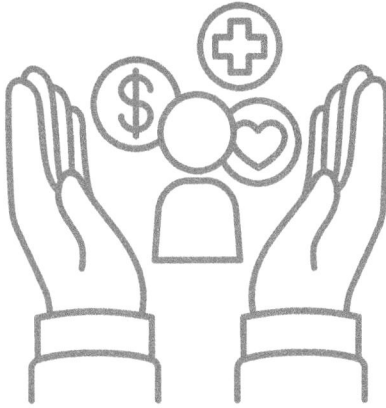

Chapter 11: The Cost of Chronic Illness

Illness is expensive. Not just money. It drains finances, energy, time, relationships, and dreams. The world often sees the disease, but it rarely sees the price tag attached to it.

Financially, it started with the doctor visits. One specialist turned into three, then five. Each visit came with a bill. Then came the tests—labs, scans, scopes, biopsies. Insurance covered some, but never all. Prescriptions piled up. Especially when I was taking twenty-two pills a day, plus weekly injections and monthly infusions. Even with coverage, the out-of-pocket costs could break anyone. And beyond the medical bills, there were hidden expenses: parking garages at hospitals, gas for long drives to appointments, food bought on the run, lost wages from time off work. Illness found a way to reach into every corner of my wallet.

But money wasn't the only cost. There was the toll on time. I spent years in waiting rooms, sometimes two to three appointments a week. My calendar was filled not with vacations, but with procedures. My kids grew used to me saying, "Mommy has a doctor's appointment." The hours added up to days, and the days to years, all spent chasing answers that often never came.

There was the emotional cost too. The guilt of missing birthdays and outings because my body couldn't keep up. The frustration of not being able to plan a simple dinner without wondering if I'd have the energy. The sting of being labeled "unreliable" when I canceled plans at the last minute, even though I wanted to be there more than anyone knew.

I'll never forget one week when I had three major appointments, each hours away. By the third trip, my gas tank and my spirit were both running on empty. I sat in the hospital parking lot and cried—not just from exhaustion, but from the sheer weight of how much being sick was stealing from my life. I felt helpless.

Then there was the price of hope. I paid in tears each time a new medication promised relief but failed. I paid in sleepless nights worrying about the future. I paid in the moments I questioned whether the doctors were making me better or slowly making me worse.

But here's the truth: while the cost of illness is steep, the value of resilience is priceless. Each bill I've paid —financial, emotional, physical—has shaped me into a woman who knows her strength, who can endure storms, and who refuses to give up. Illness has cost me so much, but it hasn't taken everything. It hasn't taken my will to fight. And that, I won't ever let it buy.

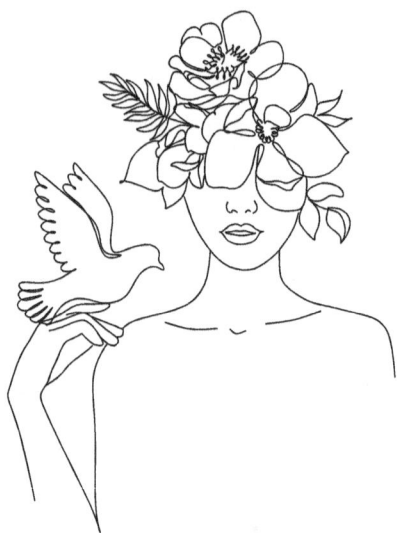

Chapter 12: Invisible Doesn't Mean Imaginary

One of the most difficult realities of living with chronic illness is that much of the struggle happens where no one can see it. My body is at war every single day—my joints ache, my skin tightens, my stomach revolts, my hands go numb, my energy drains without warning. But from the outside to someone passing me on the street or seeing me at work, I might look perfectly fine.

That disconnect creates a kind of loneliness that is hard to explain. People assume that appearance equals reality, that if you "look good," you must feel good. But the truth is, there have been countless days when I've plastered on makeup, forced a smile, and pushed through unbearable pain just to seem "normal." Those snapshots—what people see—are not the whole story.

What they don't see are the mornings I can barely drag myself out of bed. They don't see the moments when I sit in my car gathering strength just to walk into a store. They don't see the nights when I collapse into tears because my body feels like it's betraying me all over again.

I've lost count of how many times I've heard, *"But you don't look sick."* I know most people mean it kindly, but it lands like a dismissal. As if being sick should look a certain way. As if my illness isn't valid unless I look pale, frail, or hooked up to machines. Chronic illness doesn't always come with a visual marker. Sometimes the strongest battles are the ones happening silently, inside the body.

It carries a hidden cost. You're constantly deciding how much to reveal and how much to conceal. Do I tell a friend why I canceled plans again, or do I just apologize and take the blame? Do I explain to a coworker that my joints are on fire, or do I just grit my teeth and keep going? Do I risk being seen as weak, lazy, or unreliable if I tell the truth?

It wears on you. The silence, the explaining, the not being believed. There's a heavy emotional toll that comes with having to justify pain that others can't see. And when disbelief enters the picture—when people hint that you're exaggerating, or when even medical professionals dismiss what you're describing—it can make you question yourself.

But here's what I've learned: my illness doesn't need to be visible to be real. My pain is valid, my exhaustion is valid, my experience is valid—even if no one else can see it. I don't need proof to justify what I'm living through. And if you are walking this road too, neither do you.

Over time, I've also realized the importance of surrounding myself with people who get it—those who don't require evidence, who don't question my reality, who believe me simply because I said it. That kind of support is priceless.

So yes, invisible doesn't mean imaginary. It means living with battles that others may never see. It means being strong in silence, and it means giving yourself grace when the world doesn't understand. It means remembering, always, that your truth matters—even if no one else can see it.

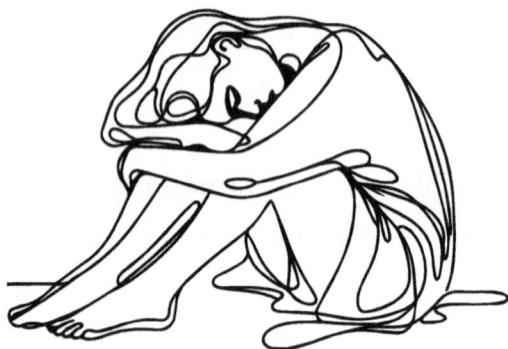

Chapter 13: The Toll on Relationships

Chronic illness doesn't just happen to the person living with it—it happens to everyone around them. It seeps into family, friendships, and partnerships, testing bonds in ways I never expected.

At first, I tried to protect the people I loved. I downplayed my pain, smiled when I was exhausted, and said "I'm fine" more often than I should have. But illness has a way of showing itself, no matter how hard you try to hide it. Eventually, the cracks appeared, and every relationship around me had to shift.

Some relationships grew stronger. The people who

truly cared leaned in closer. They learned patience, accepted cancellations, and stood by me even when I couldn't give them the same energy back.

I'll never forget the night I had to cancel plans with a close friend for the third time in a row. I texted, ashamed, waiting for the disappointment. Instead, she replied: "Don't worry, I'll come sit with you instead." She showed up with snacks and we watched TV together. No expectations, no pressure—just presence. That's love in action.

Others drifted away. Not everyone could handle the unpredictability. Some didn't know what to say, so they said nothing. It hurt, but I've come to understand that illness has a way of revealing who your people truly are.

Romantic relationships carried their own weight. Illness brings a vulnerability that is hard to share— admitting limits, asking for help, exposing fears.

Parenting, too, was shaped by my illness. My children have seen more than I ever wanted them to. I worried they'd remember me only as the sick mom, the one who couldn't always keep up. But what they've seen is resilience. They've learned compassion, patience, and strength—not from lectures, but from watching me fight to keep going.

Friendships had to be redefined. Gone were the long nights out and spontaneous plans. In their place came shorter visits, quiet conversations, and messages that meant more than grand gestures ever could. The friends who stayed became more precious than ever.

Illness reshaped every connection in my life. Some bonds cracked under the pressure. Others grew roots so deep they'll never break. And while I grieve the losses, I'm grateful for the love that has endured. Love that adapts, bends, and shows up even when life doesn't go as planned.

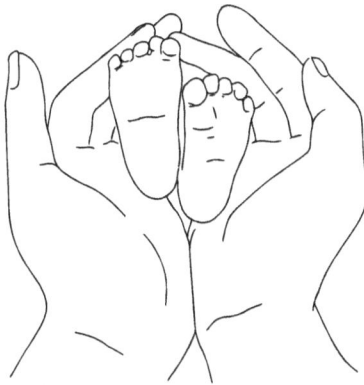

Chapter 14: Parenting with a Chronic Illness

Motherhood has always been a part of who I am, but living with a chronic illness changed how I thought it would look. I pictured staying up late for movie nights, cooking big family meals without a second thought. Instead, I found myself balancing motherhood with the reality of a body that doesn't always cooperate.

Parenting with chronic illnesses means carrying guilt alongside love. There are days I can't keep up, days when pain forces me to say no, days when fatigue steals the energy I wanted to give them. I've missed school events. I've had to cancel plans. I've worried that my kids would feel like they were missing out

One night, my child asked me why I always seemed so tired. I froze, unsure how to explain something so big in words they'd understand. I finally said, "My body works harder than it should, even when I'm resting. That's why I get tired quicker." They nodded and hugged me, and in that moment, I realized they didn't need perfection—they just needed me.

In those same moments, I've seen something remarkable. My children have grown into people with a depth of compassion and resilience that humbles me. They've watched me fight, and in that, they've learned what strength really looks like. They know that love isn't measured in activities or perfection—it's measured in presence, in showing up even when it's hard.

Illness reshaped the way I mother, but it didn't take away my ability to love fiercely. Instead, it forced me to redefine it. I've learned to be creative in how I connect with my kids: shorter outings, quieter moments, and time that's meaningful, even if it doesn't look like what I once imagined.

I've also learned to accept help, something that never came easily to me. Allowing others to step in when I couldn't, was hard at first—it felt like failure. But I see now that it doesn't mean I'm less of a mother. It means my children are surrounded by a community of love, and that is its own kind of blessing.

Parenting with a chronic illness is messy and imperfect. There are tears, both theirs and mine. But there is also laughter, tenderness, and moments I'll never forget. My illness may shape the way I mother, but it has never diminished the love I carry for my children. If anything, it's made that love burn brighter —because I know how precious every moment really is.

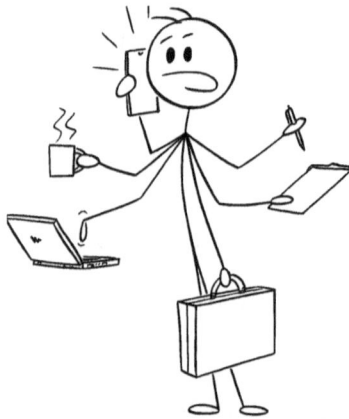

Chapter 15: Back to Work, Back to Life

I spent a few years recovering—not from healing, but from the weight of it all. The constant appointments, the endless pills, the cycle of being treated but never feeling better. For a while, I stepped away from work entirely, trying to focus on managing my health.

But staying home all the time made me feel like I was waiting to die. I was sick of being sick, sick of staring at the same walls, sick of my world shrinking smaller, and smaller. I realized that even if my pain didn't disappear, I couldn't let it consume everything. I needed to move, to live, to feel like me again.

So, I went back to work.

I didn't return to an office or a job with predictable hours—I went back to bartending. Work that demands energy, speed, and social interaction. On paper, it made no sense. My body was still in pain every day. Some shifts stretched me to my limits. But something in me knew I needed it.

Behind the bar, I wasn't just a patient. I wasn't defined by pills or diagnoses. I was Jeanette again laughing with customers, moving through the rhythm of busy nights, finding strength in the hustle. Even when my legs felt heavy or my wrists screamed in pain, I kept pushing. Because for me, still moving meant still living.

One especially busy night, my legs ached so badly I thought I might collapse. I wanted to walk out, go home, crawl into bed. But then a regular customer caught my eye, raised a glass, and said, "You always brighten this place." That reminder—that I was more than my illness—carried me through the shift.

Some days were brutal. There were moments I wanted to crawl into bed and cry like I used to. But I didn't. I kept going. And strangely, that movement helped—because the less I moved, the stiffer I got.

a Day in my Life

Chapter 16: A Day in My Life

From the outside, my day may look ordinary. But every hour is shaped by illness, even in ways others don't notice.

Mornings are the hardest. My alarm rings, but my body refuses to cooperate. My joints ache, my hands feel stiff, and just swinging my legs out of bed takes effort. What used to take fifteen minutes—showering, dressing, getting ready—now takes an hour or more. By the time I'm dressed, I already feel like I've run a marathon.

Breakfast isn't simple either. Because of gastroparesis and Barrett's esophagus, food is no longer just food —it's calculation. Will this upset my stomach? Will this trigger reflux? Will I regret this meal in an hour? Some mornings I drink my nutrition instead of eating it, because chewing and swallowing feels like too much.

Then comes work.

Bartending isn't the easiest job for someone with chronic illness, but I chose it because I needed to keep moving. Sitting at home waiting for answers felt like waiting to die. At the bar, I keep busy, I smile, I connect with people. What most don't see is the pain hidden behind that smile. They don't notice when my hands tremble as I twist open a bottle, or when my feet swell after standing for hours.

By the time I clock out, my body is begging for rest. I drive home in silence, too exhausted for music. I want to collapse the second I walk in the door, but I keep going because life doesn't pause. Dinner for the kids, checking homework, tidying the house. Finally, when the house is quiet, I let myself exhale.

But even nights aren't restful. Pain doesn't care that it's bedtime. Some nights I fall asleep quickly, other nights I toss and turn until the clock hits 3 a.m., my mind buzzing and my body aching. When I finally drift off, it's with the knowledge that I'll do it all again tomorrow.

This is a day in my life. Ordinary and extraordinary all at once. Harder than it looks, but filled with love that makes every struggle worth it.

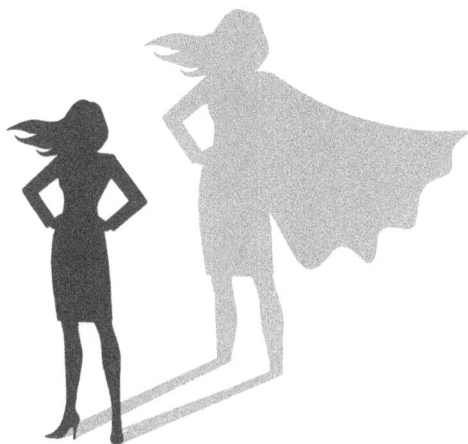

Chapter 17: Redefining Strength

Before illness, I thought I knew what strength was. Strength meant powering through long days without stopping. It meant taking care of everyone else before myself. It meant carrying heavy loads, never asking for help, and never showing weakness.

Illness stripped away that version of strength. My body forced me to slow down, to acknowledge limits I didn't want to admit were there. At first, I felt like I had failed. If I couldn't keep up, if I couldn't do everything I once could—was I still strong?

Over time, I realized strength had to be redefined. Strength was no longer about how much I could do— it was about how I kept going, even when I could do less.

Strength became quieter. It became getting out of bed on mornings when my body felt like lead. It became saying, "I can't," even when I hated the words. It became asking for help, even when my pride screamed not to.

One morning, I couldn't open a jar of pasta sauce. I twisted and twisted until my hands throbbed, then finally set it down in defeat. My son came over, picked it up, and popped it open easily. I laughed, but inside I was crushed. That jar reminded me that strength doesn't always look like brute force. That night, I realized true strength was letting myself laugh instead of cry.

Strength is not about invincibility—it's about vulnerability. It's showing up in the middle of the struggle, not after it's gone. It's admitting the pain but refusing to let it win.

There is strength in the quiet moments—in tears that

fall but don't break you, in resting even when the world calls it weakness, in showing love to others even when your own body is heavy with pain.

Illness has taught me that true strength is not loud, flashy, or visible to the world. It's quiet. Steady. Resilient. It bends, but it doesn't break. And the fact that I am still here, still fighting, still choosing to live —that is strength in its purest form.

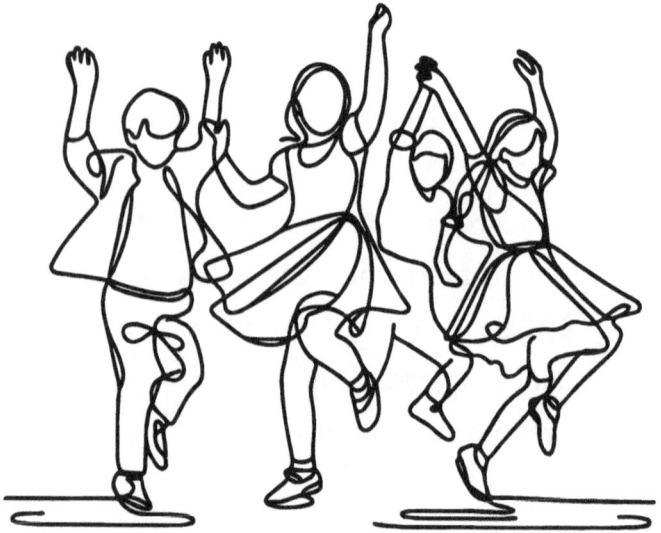

Chapter 18: Joy Still Exists

When you first hear the words *chronic illness,* joy feels like it vanishes. The weight of symptoms, the endless appointments, the constant uncertainty—it all overshadows the simple pleasures you once took for granted. For a while, I thought joy was gone for good.

But slowly, I realized joy wasn't gone—it had simply changed shape.

Joy stopped being about big, extravagant moments. Instead, it started showing up in smaller, quieter places. In the sound of my children's laughter. In the warmth of the sun on my skin during a rare good morning. In finishing a work shift I thought I couldn't get through. In drinking coffee without wincing from reflux.

Living with illness taught me to notice things I used to overlook. I no longer assume tomorrow will feel like today, so I hold tighter to the good moments when they come. Those flashes of relief, comfort, or happiness become treasures—reminders that pain isn't the only story my body tells.

One afternoon, I sat outside, wrapped in a blanket, sipping tea. For the first time in weeks, the pain was lighter. The breeze touched my skin, and I felt tears well up—not from sadness, but from gratitude. That tiny moment of peace felt like a miracle.

Joy is also deeply tied to gratitude. Gratitude for the people who stand by me. Gratitude for the community of others living with autoimmune diseases who remind me I'm not alone. Gratitude for myself, for continuing to fight even when the road is long and unfair. For my own strength on the days, I thought I had none.

This doesn't mean every day is joyful. Some days are dark. Some days I collapse in exhaustion or frustration. But even in those seasons, joy doesn't disappear—it waits. Sometimes quietly. Sometimes stubbornly. But it's still there, waiting to be found.

That is the lesson illness gave me about joy: it doesn't vanish in hardship. It bends. It hides. It shifts. And when I do find it, it feels even more powerful—because I know how much it means to feel it at all.

Joy still exists. And when I choose to see it, it makes all the difference.

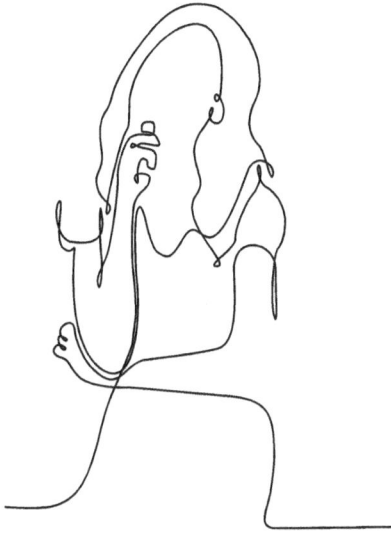

Chapter 19: What I Wish People Knew

Living with chronic illness has shown me how invisible suffering can be. I've carried pain, exhaustion, and fear in silence, all while smiling on the outside. And while I've grown stronger in my own way, there are things I wish people could see—things I wish they understood.

I wish people knew how exhausting it is just to exist.

This fatigue is not ordinary tiredness. It's not something that a good night's sleep can fix. It's a deep, bone-crushing exhaustion that clings to me no matter what I do. Some days, simply getting dressed feels like running a marathon.

I wish people knew how much effort goes into pretending.

I've become skilled at covering up my pain with a smile, at saying "I'm fine" when the truth would take too much explaining. Pretending takes energy, but sometimes it feels easier than being misunderstood.

I wish people knew how unpredictable my life is.

I can wake up one morning with hope for the day, and by afternoon be knocked down by pain or fatigue. This unpredictability makes me cancel plans, leave early, or sometimes disappear without warning. It's not a lack of care—it's my reality.

I wish people knew I don't need to be fixed.

I don't need miracle cures pulled from the internet. I don't need comparisons to someone's cousin who "got better." What I need is compassion, patience, and presence. Sometimes the greatest gift is a simple, "I believe you."

Above all, I wish people knew that I am still me. Illness has changed parts of my life, yes, but it hasn't erased who I am. I still dream. I still laugh. I still love deeply. I am not just a diagnosis—I am a whole person who happens to carry battles you can't see.

If you love someone with a chronic illness, believe them. Trust them. Offer grace. Sometimes the greatest gift isn't a cure—it's compassion.

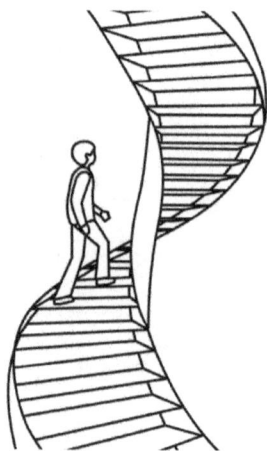

Chapter 20: Healing Isn't Linear

When I was first diagnosed, I thought if I did everything right—took the medications, went to every appointment, followed the doctors' instructions—then healing would be steady. I imagined it as a staircase: one step up, then another, until eventually I'd reach the top.

But chronic illness doesn't work like that. Healing isn't a staircase. It's a winding road, full of detours, setbacks, and loops that bring you back to places you thought you'd already left behind.

There are days when I wake up and feel almost normal. Days when the pain is lighter, when my energy is a little stronger, when I think, maybe I've turned a corner. But then there are flares. Without warning, the fatigue crushes me again, my joints lock, my skin tightens, and I find myself right back in survival mode. The rhythm of progress and relapse can be brutal.

At first, those setbacks felt like failures. I'd think, *What's the point of trying if I just keep ending up here again?* I grieved every backslide as if it erased the progress I had made.

Over time, though, I've learned that this is simply the nature of healing. It's not a straight line—it's a rhythm of rising and falling. The good days don't cancel out the hard ones, and the hard days don't erase the progress I've made. Both are part of the story.

Healing, I've realized, is not about reaching an endpoint. It's about learning to live fully, even when the illness doesn't go away. It's about celebrating the small victories—a meal enjoyed without pain, a shift finished at work, a morning when I could walk without stiffness. It's about giving myself grace on the days when I can't do much at all.

The truth is, there may never be a "cure" for me. But there is a way to live, to hope, and to keep moving forward—even if the road bends and twists along the way.

Healing isn't linear. But it's still healing. Every time I choose to rise again, even after a setback, I'm moving forward—whether the world can see it or not.

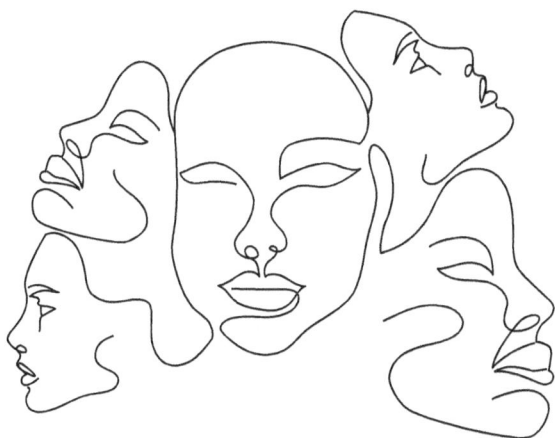

Chapter 21: Worlds Within Me

There are worlds inside me that no one else can see.

There is the world of my body—aching, stiff, unpredictable. A world where joints swell, skin tightens, blood vessels constrict, and fatigue presses down like a weight I cannot set aside. It is a world of limits, of medications and procedures, of learning how to live within boundaries I never asked for.

There is the world of my mind—restless, questioning, sometimes overwhelmed. A world filled with endless what-ifs: *Why me? How long? Will it get worse?* But also filled with quiet answers I didn't know I carried: *Because you are strong. Because you will endure. Because you will find a way forward.*

There is the world of my heart—wounded but still beating with hope. A world where love fuels me, where laughter breaks through even the heaviest pain, where gratitude blooms in the smallest corners of my days. My heart clings to light, even when darkness tries to take over.

And there is the world of my spirit—soft, but unshakable. A world that whispers to me in the stillness: *You are still here. You are still you.*

I remember lying awake one night, staring at the ceiling, feeling like my body was failing me in every possible way. My mind spiraled with fear; my heart ached with grief. But then, somewhere deep inside, my spirit whispered: "You're still here. That's enough." And it was. That small reminder carried me through another day.

Sometimes, these worlds collide. The body overwhelms the mind. The mind drowns the heart. The heart struggles to lift the spirit. But other times, these worlds hold each other together—the spirit strengthens the body, the heart steadies the mind, and somehow, I rise again.

I have learned that living with chronic illness means carrying all of these worlds at once. Some are heavy, some are light. Some are filled with pain, others with beauty. Together, they make me who I am.

The outside world may never see them, but I do. And maybe that's the truest strength of all—to know the worlds within me, and to keep living fully inside them.

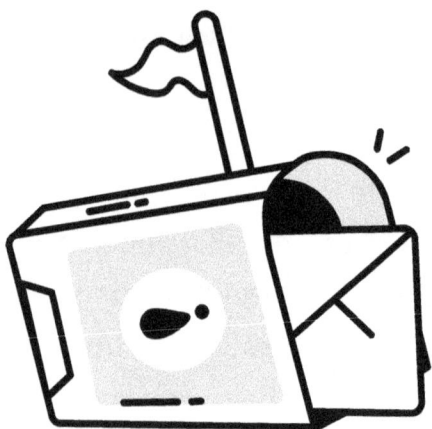

Chapter 22: Letters I Never Sent

To the Doctor Who Didn't Listen

You saw me, but you didn't *see* me. You looked at my lab results, checked boxes, and rushed through explanations, but you never looked into my eyes long enough to notice the pain that lived there. When I tried to tell you my symptoms, you brushed me off. When I begged you to listen, you acted like I was exaggerating.

Do you know what that did to me? It made me question myself. It made me wonder if I was crazy, if maybe I was imagining it all. But the pain was real. The exhaustion was real. The fear was real. And your dismissal didn't make it disappear—it only added another layer of suffering.

To My Younger Self, Right Before Diagnosis

Sweet girl, you have no idea what's about to come. Right now you're living life with a rhythm you think will last forever—busy days, long nights, laughter with your kids, dreams that feel wide open. You don't know yet that your body is about to change the rules.

You will soon hear words you never expected: scleroderma, lupus, autoimmune, chronic, incurable. Those words will feel like thunder crashing down. You will cry. You will rage. You will grieve the life you thought was yours. There will be days when you feel like giving up, nights when you wonder how you'll keep going.

But listen to me—you will keep going. You will

discover strength you never imagined. You'll learn that your body may break down, but your spirit won't. You'll find new ways to live, new ways to love, new ways to fight. You'll lose people who don't understand, but you'll also find community in places you never expected.

Hold onto hope, even when it feels fragile. Trust that even through pain, joy will find you. And never forget —you are more than a diagnosis.

To My Children

My loves, my reasons for breathing—there are so many things I want you to know. I know my illness has stolen moments from us. I know you've seen me in pain when you should've only seen me laughing. I know there were times I had to say "not today" when all I wanted was to say "yes."

But please know this: every decision I made, every rest I took, every appointment I went to—it was all because I wanted to be here with you longer. I wanted to fight for time, for milestones, for memories we still have yet to make.

You are the reason I wake up even when I don't want to. You are the reason I smile through tears, work when I'm exhausted, and keep pushing when my body begs me to stop. When you see me tired, don't mistake it for weakness. Know that it's proof of how much I love you—because even in my weakest moments, I keep going for you.

Someday, when you face your own storms, I hope you remember this: strength doesn't always look like power. Sometimes it looks like persistence. And if you ever wonder what love looks like, I hope you think of me—fighting, stumbling, but never giving up, because my heart beats for you.

To My Family

To my family—my anchors in this storm, my steady place when everything else feels uncertain.

I know this illness hasn't just touched me—it has touched all of you. You've watched me struggle, sometimes powerless to help. You've carried me when I was too weak to carry myself, both literally and figuratively. And I know it hasn't been easy.

I've seen the worry in your eyes when you thought I wasn't looking. I've felt the tension in your voices when another flare kept me in bed or another hospital stay rearranged everyone's plans. I know my illness has disrupted holidays, birthdays, and everyday life. For that, I carry guilt—but I also carry gratitude. Because through all the detours and delays, you stayed.

Thank you for the patience you showed on days when I snapped out of pain or exhaustion. Thank you for the rides to appointments, the meals cooked, the errands run when I couldn't get up. Thank you for believing me when others doubted, for reminding me I wasn't "crazy" when doctors made me question myself.

You may never fully understand how much your presence has saved me. Even in silence, your support has been medicine I couldn't get from a pharmacy.

This illness may have changed what I can do, but it hasn't changed my love for you. If anything, it's deepened it. Because I've seen firsthand how strong and selfless my family can be. You are the reason I keep choosing to fight. You are the net that catches me when I fall. And though I can't always show it the way I want to, please know that every breath I take in this fight is also a love letter to you.

To My Disease

You barged into my life without warning. You took things from me I can never get back—energy, freedom, certainty. You tried to make me smaller, weaker, less alive.

But here's what you don't understand: you may live in my body, but you don't own my spirit. You may change the way I move through the world, but you cannot take away my will to keep moving. You may have stolen my comfort, but you will never steal my courage.

Yes, you've broken me down. But in those cracks, light still shines through. You've made me cry rivers, but those tears have watered strength I didn't know I had.

You thought you could silence me, but instead you've made me louder.

You will always be part of my story—but you don't get to write the ending. That belongs to me. And I choose to end it with defiance, with resilience, and with love.

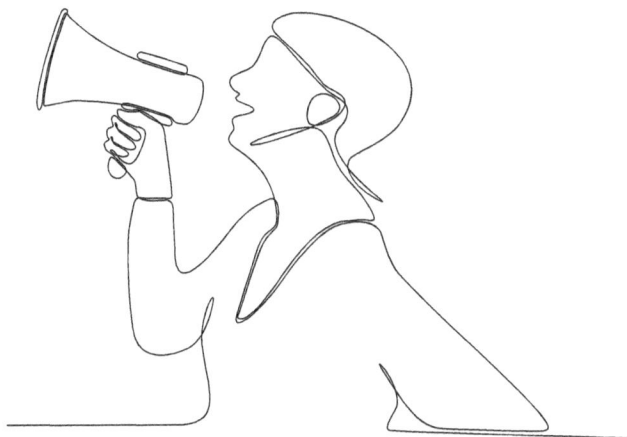

Chapter 23: Why I Speak Up

For a long time, I stayed quiet. I trusted the doctors to lead, let friends assume I was fine, and hid my pain behind polite smiles. Silence felt safer. If I didn't speak up, I couldn't be brushed off, doubted, or misunderstood.

But silence has its own cost. It weighs heavy. It makes you feel invisible. And I realized one day that if I didn't use my voice, my story would disappear into the shadows—along with all the others who never got the chance to be heard.

So, I began to speak.

At first, it was shaky. I asked questions at appointments instead of nodding along. I told friends "I can't" instead of pretending. I shared pieces of my journey publicly, even when it scared me. Each time, I felt vulnerable. But each time, I also felt a little freer. My truth was no longer trapped inside me.

I still remember the first time I posted openly about my illness online. My hands trembled as I hit "share." I worried people would pity me, or worse, ignore me. But then the comments started to come— "Me too." "I thought I was alone." That day, I realized my voice wasn't just mine—it was a bridge.

And the more I spoke, the more I understood: my voice is NOT just mine. It belongs to the people who feel silenced in their own illness. To the patients dismissed by doctors. To the ones who are told *"you don't look sick."* To the ones who scroll online in the middle of the night searching for someone—anyone —who understands.

The Heart of Advocacy

My voice became more than words.

It became defiance.

It became survival.

It became a bridge to others walking this same hard road.

Advocacy doesn't mean I have all the answers. It doesn't mean I'm fearless. It means I refuse to let this disease define the narrative alone. It means I share my truth in hopes that someone else will see themselves in it, and know they are not alone.

I speak up because awareness matters. Because every story told makes it harder for the world to ignore us. Because maybe one day, a doctor will listen more closely, research will go further, and someone else's journey will be a little lighter.

But most of all, I speak up because I can. Because I'm still here. And as long as I'm still here, I refuse to stay silent.

A Letter to the Newly Diagnosed

Dear Warrior,

If you are reading this, it means your world has just shifted. Maybe you've been told you have scleroderma, MCTD, lupus, or another illness that sounds foreign and overwhelming. I know what you're feeling—the fear, the confusion, the late-night questions you can't stop asking.

I've been there. I remember sitting in sterile offices, staring at paperwork filled with words I didn't understand, wondering if my life as I knew it was already over. I remember the loneliness, the anger, the silent grief of realizing my body would never be the same.

So, I want to tell you what I wish someone had told me:

You are not alone.

This disease may be rare, but you are not the only one fighting it. There is a community of people who are battling similar wars.

It's okay to grieve.

You are losing the version of yourself you once knew, and that hurts. Let yourself feel it. Grief isn't weakness—it's part of the process of learning to live again.

You are still you.

Illness will change your routines, your energy, and maybe even your plans. But it cannot erase who you are at your core—your love, your humor, your creativity, your strength.

Your strength will surprise you.

There will be days when you think you can't keep going—and then you will. Every time you rise after being knocked down, you will discover a resilience you didn't know you had.

This isn't the end of your story.

It's the start of a new chapter. One that may be harder, yes—but also one that will reveal parts of yourself you never knew existed.

After my diagnosis, I sat awake night after night, scrolling forums, desperate to find someone who understood. When I finally did, when I saw someone put my feelings into words, I cried with relief. You will find those people, too. And you will discover that hope is contagious.

The road ahead won't be easy. There will be setbacks, flares, and moments when you question everything. But there will also be victories, laughter, love, and days you will hold onto with gratitude.

So, take it one step at a time. Celebrate the small wins. Rest when you need to. Speak up when you aren't being heard. And above all, know this: you are stronger than this disease, and your story is far from over.

With love, solidarity, and hope,
Jeanette

Epilogue: I'm Still Here

I've faced pain that shook me to my core. I've been given diagnoses that tried to strip away my hope. I've lost pieces of the life I thought I'd have, and I've grieved more than I ever thought possible.

And yet—through it all—I'm still here.

Still here, waking up each morning, no matter how heavy the day feels.
Still here, pushing forward even when my body resists.
Still here, showing up for my children, my loved ones, and myself.
Still here, choosing life even in the middle of struggle.

There are days when I come home from work, body aching, eyes burning with exhaustion, and I collapse onto the couch. For a moment, I think, "I can't do this anymore." And then I hear my daughter's laughter from the other room, or my son's voice on the phone, and I remember exactly why I keep going.

My scars, my fatigue, my limits—they are not signs of weakness. They are proof of survival. They are reminders that illness did not win. I don't know what tomorrow will bring. None of us do. But I know that as long as I have breath in my body, I will keep speaking, keep loving, and keep living as fully as I can.

If you are holding this book, know this: you are still here, too. And that means your story isn't finished.

Hold on. Keep going. Let yourself cry when you need to, rest when you must, and rise again when you can. Strength doesn't mean being unbreakable—it means refusing to give up, even when the world tries to break you.

I'm Jeanette.
I'm still me.
And most importantly—**I'm still here.**

Glossary of Terms

Autoimmune Disease A condition in which the immune system mistakenly attacks the body's own tissues, leading to inflammation and damage.

Barrett's Esophagus A complication of chronic acid reflux (GERD) where the lining of the esophagus changes, tightens, and erodes, increasing the risk of cancer.

Chronic Illness A long-term health condition that often has no cure and must be managed over time.

Epidemiology The study of how diseases affect populations, including risk factors and prevention.

Epstein-Barr Virus (EBV) A common virus that can cause mononucleosis ("mono"). It has also been linked to triggering some autoimmune diseases.

Flares Periods when symptoms suddenly worsen or become more severe. Common in autoimmune conditions.

Gastroparesis A digestive condition where the stomach muscles don't work properly, slowing or stopping the movement of food into the small intestine.

IBD (Inflammatory Bowel Disease) A group of conditions (including Crohn's disease and ulcerative colitis) that cause chronic inflammation of the digestive tract.

Infusion A medical treatment where medication is delivered directly into the bloodstream through an IV.

Lupus (Systemic Lupus Erythematosus, SLE) A chronic autoimmune disease where the immune system attacks the skin, joints, kidneys, and other organs.

Mixed Connective Tissue Disease (MCTD) An overlap autoimmune disorder that combines features of lupus, scleroderma, rheumatoid arthritis, and more.

Methotrexate A medication originally developed for cancer that is also used at lower doses to treat autoimmune diseases.

Rheumatoid Arthritis (RA) An autoimmune disease where the immune system attacks the joints, causing pain, swelling, and damage.

Raynaud's Phenomenon A condition that affects blood flow, often in the fingers and toes, triggered by cold or stress. It causes them to turn white, blue, purple, and then red as blood flow returns, painfully.

Remission A period during which symptoms decrease or disappear.

Scleroderma A rare autoimmune disease that causes hardening and tightening of the skin and connective tissues, and can affect internal organs.

Specialist A doctor who focuses on a specific area of medicine, such as rheumatology (joints/autoimmune), gastroenterology (digestive system), or dermatology (skin).

Steroids (Corticosteroids) Medications that reduce inflammation and suppress the immune system. Often used for flares.

Support Group A community of patients and caregivers who share experiences, resources, and encouragement.

Systemic Sclerosis Formerly known as CREST syndrome. CREST is an acronym for the five main features of a limited form of scleroderma: **C**alcinosis, **R**aynaud's phenomenon, **E**sophophageal dysfunction, **S**clerodactyly, and **T**elangiectasia. It is an autoimmune connective tissue disorder that causes hardening and tightening of the skin and connective tissues.

Helpful Resources

LUPUS

• Lupus Foundation of America – National Resource Center on Lupus (education, support, community): *https://www.lupus.org*

• Lupus Research Alliance (research updates, advocacy): *https://www.lupusresearch.org*

• HSS LupusLine & support programs (free peer support, multilingual resources): *https://www.hss.edu/lupus-programs.asp*

• American College of Rheumatology – Patient info on lupus: *https://rheumatology.org/patients/lupus*

• NIAMS/NIH – Lupus overview & treatment: *https://www.niams.nih.gov/health-topics/lupus*

• CDC – Lupus education & health tips: *https://www.cdc.gov/lupus*

SCLERODERMA

• National Scleroderma Foundation (support groups, education, community): *https://scleroderma.org*   117

• Scleroderma Research Foundation (research, patient education): https://srfcure.org

• Johns Hopkins Scleroderma Center (patient resources, clinical expertise): https://www.hopkinsscleroderma.org

• Boston University Scleroderma Program (care & research): https://www.bumc.bu.edu/scleroderma

• American College of Rheumatology – Patient info on scleroderma: https://rheumatology.org/patients/scleroderma

• NIAMS/NIH – Scleroderma overview: https://www.niams.nih.gov/health-topics/scleroderma

RHEUMATOID ARTHRITIS (RA)

• Arthritis Foundation (resources, tools, local events & connect groups): https://www.arthritis.org

• American College of Rheumatology – Patient info on RA: https://rheumatology.org/patients/rheumatoid-arthritis

• Rheumatoid Arthritis Foundation (Help Fight RA) – education & support: *https://www.helpfightra.org*

• CreakyJoints (patient community, practical guides): *https://creakyjoints.org*

• NIAMS/NIH – RA overview & treatment options: *https://www.niams.nih.gov/health-topics/rheumatoid-arthritis*

• Hospital for Special Surgery (HSS) – RA education hub: *https://www.hss.edu/condition-list_rheumatoid-arthritis.asp*

GASTROPARESIS

• G-PACT (Gastroparesis Patient Association for Cures & Treatments): *https://www.g-pact.org*

• IFFGD (International Foundation for Gastrointestinal Disorders) – Gastroparesis info: *https://aboutgastroparesis.org* main: *https://iffgd.org*

- NIDDK/NIH – Gastroparesis overview: https://www.niddk.nih.gov/health-information/digestive-diseases/gastroparesis

- AGA (American Gastroenterological Association) – Patient info: https://gastro.org/patient-care/patient-info

- Oley Foundation (tube feeding/TPN support, nutrition resources): https://oley.org

IBD (CROHN'S DISEASE & ULCERATIVE COLITIS)

- Crohn's & Colitis Foundation – IBD Help Center, education & support: https://www.crohnscolitisfoundation.org

- CDC – IBD information & resources: https://www.cdc.gov/ibd

- NIDDK/NIH – IBD overview (Crohn's & UC): https://www.niddk.nih.gov/health-information/digestive-diseases/inflammatory-bowel-disease

- ImproveCareNow (pediatric/teen IBD care network): *https://www.improvecarenow.org*

- UChicago Medicine IBD Center – patient education & support groups: *https://www.uchicagomedicine.org/conditions-services/inflammatory-bowel-disease*

RAYNAUD'S PHENOMENON

- Raynaud's Association – education, coping tips, community: *https://www.raynauds.org*

- American College of Rheumatology – Raynaud's patient info: *https://rheumatology.org/patients/raynauds-phenomenon*

- NIAMS/NIH – Raynaud's overview: *https://www.niams.nih.gov/health-topics/raynauds-phenomenon*

- National Scleroderma Foundation – Raynaud's resources & warming strategies: *https://scleroderma.org (search "Raynaud's" on site)*

GENERAL SUPPORT: FINANCIAL AID, ADVOCACY, CLINICAL TRIALS

- Patient Advocate Foundation (case management, insurance help, co-pay relief): *https://www.patientadvocate.org*

- PAN Foundation (co-pay & premium assistance for eligible conditions): *https://www.panfoundation.org*

- NeedyMeds (drug discount cards, assistance program directory): *https://www.needymeds.org*

- ClinicalTrials.gov (search trials by condition): *https://clinicaltrials.gov*

- 211 (local services: transportation, food, housing support) – Dial 211 or visit *https://www.211.org*

- Mental Health: 988 Suicide & Crisis Lifeline (free, 24/7): Call or text 988; chat at *https://988lifeline.org*

Tips for Readers

If you've made it this far, thank you — not just for reading my story, but for allowing yourself to connect with it. Whether you're living with an autoimmune or chronic illness, love someone who is, or simply needed a reminder that strength doesn't always look like "doing it all," I hope these words stay with you.

• Give yourself permission to rest. Your worth isn't measured by how productive you are. Healing requires gentleness, not guilt.

• Advocate for yourself, even when your voice shakes. You know your body best. Don't be afraid to ask questions or say, "something isn't right."

• Celebrate small victories. Getting out of bed, making it to an appointment, or even just taking a shower on a hard day — those are wins worth acknowledging.

• Protect your energy. You can love people deeply and still choose peace over explaining yourself.

• Don't compare your healing to anyone else's. This journey is yours. There's no timeline, no finish line, no "perfect" recovery.

• Find joy in the in-between moments. A laugh that surprises you, a sunset that quiets your mind, or a song that speaks your heart — they're all medicine, too.

• Remember: You are not your illness. You are strength, softness, courage, and grace all wrapped into one.

• And on the days it feels too heavy — remind yourself: You are still here.
And that alone is everything.

*** *Always verify support group schedules and insurance/assistance eligibility on each site.*

*** *Bring printed PDFs or links from these sites to appointments to help guide conversations with your care team.*

www.ingramcontent.com/pod-product-compliance
Lightning Source LLC
Chambersburg PA
CBHW031436270326
41930CB00007B/741